Hospice – A Holistic Journey Through the Shadow of Death
A Dissertation

James W. Strickland, LCSW, PhD

Outskirts Press, Inc.
Denver, Colorado

Acknowledgements

I owe everything I am and everything I have achieved in life to my deceased mother and father, Mary G. and Cledies. They were the inspiration for all that I've accomplished on this plane. I am eternally indebted to my wife, Janyce, my children, Gina, Richie and Roderick who supported my dreams through the years at the sacrifice of some of their own desires. They were always there when I had my head in a book or left them after work to attend classes. I am also indebted to my brother in law, Reverend Frank Burton and my big sister Dorothy Burton who called me "Doc" and promoted my desire to aspire to that spiritual and scholastic height.

I thank friends like Nancy Sivak, Sandra Eller, Bennie Stephens, Dr. Ram B. Singh, Linda Tuber, Angela Williams, Dr. Levester Lyons, Dr. Frankie B. Calloway and so many other friends, family and colleagues who inspired me to move forward and follow my dreams. I owe a debt of gratitude to Leslie West and Annette Reynolds, my AIHT Faculty Advisors for coaching me on this journey and providing technical guidance and scholarly advice. Last but not least, I thank all the hospices in the world for their compassionate care for mankind during the end of life in this space.

Abstract

Hospice – A Holistic Journey through the Shadow of Death

James W Strickland

This paper presents a journey through the end of life accompanied by caregivers who believe in the inner strength of the traveler. Interdisciplinary Team descriptions of the patient's preparations for death are noted. The paper demonstrates how hospice staff in a rural community tunes into the patient's emotional state to make the transition from a full life to the end of life a heart rendering and memorable event. Survey results from Doctors, Nurses and Hospice care team members demonstrate that hospice provides a holistic approach to end of life care.

Table of Contents

Chapter 1
Hospice

The survey of a hospice team in a rural community showed how the team tuned into the dying patient's emotional states in order to make their transition from a full life through end of life a heart rendering and compassionate event. Hospice is a service provided patients receiving specialized care not to cure but to treat in a humanistic and compassionate manner during the end stages of life. Hospice was approved as a Medicare provider in 1982 and through this approval; it became more accessible to families regardless of the ability to pay. The goal is to insure the patient is as comfortable as possible and free of pain. Another goal is to insure the patient is treated humanely and given the utmost respect in order that the patient can live the rest of his/her life in a familiar environment. In a home environment, the patient can continue to practice and observe any spiritual or cultural belief system without prejudice.

Chapter 2
Origin of Hospice

According to Callanan and Kelley, Dr. Cicely Saunders made the statement, "You matter because you are." (Callanan and Kelley, 25) In this statement she reminded her dying patients that they mattered to the end of their lives. In 1967 she opened the St. Christopher's Hospice in London and worked with physicians and nurses to assist their dying patients with empathetic and compassionate care. These earlier works formed the basis of worldwide hospices as we know them today.

Hospice was first introduced to America by Doctor Saunders during a visit to Yale University. She gave lectures on treatment of the terminally ill to care providers including physicians, nurses, clergy, social workers and volunteers. Hospice can turn death from a cold impersonal experience into a service where patients can die at home. (Kessler, 2007). In addition to palliative care, hospice provides much needed bereavement, spiritual and grief counseling services to the family survivors. When administered properly, professionally and ethically; hospice can prove to be a cost effective service as it keeps the dying patient out of the hospital where he/she would still be provided curative care when no cure is expected. Hospice in some cities is run as a business and competes for the dying just like funeral homes. It is this reason that families of the dying patient should be well informed of their rights and the patient's rights. Unfortunately, when the patient enrolls in hospice emotions run too high for some families to investigate patient's rights. Someone in the family or the hospital system should step up to the plate and act as a patient advocate.

Chapter 3
The Nearing Death Experience

Kathleen Dowling Singh says the nearing death experience often seems to confer a special kind of knowledge, a quality of knowing. (Singh, 10) The dying person has the internal knowledge that no one around him/her is able to understand. The energies that were once used to stay alive are now turned into spiritual energies that are connecting with the unknown realm of a new self. Sometimes these energies can be felt by persons surrounding the dying individual. In questioning families of the dying, they indicated that they felt a sudden rush of warm air or a sudden coolness in the room during their dying relative's transition from life to death. There is no evidence found in the literature as to what caused these sudden changes in atmosphere in the room of the dying person.

Chapter 4
Hospice in Rural Areas

Hospice in small town rural areas can be different from those located in large cities. There are many obstacles that have to be surmounted in the care of dying patients and families in rural areas. Transportation is a major obstacle. The lack of public transportation places the greatest barrier between the patient and the caregivers. Oftentimes the hospice team has to travel distances of 50 miles or more through muddy and unpaved country roads. There are times when hospice vehicles get bogged down in the mud and slide off narrow rain slickened roads. Tow trucks have to be summoned and in the rural areas they are not readily available. Valuable time is often lost and this time away from the patient can be critical in administering much needed pain medications or oxygen. Improperly wired homes also pose a major problem. Beds, oxygen equipment and pain pumps all use electricity and some must be used simultaneously. Improperly wired homes don't always allow for all the necessary equipment to operate at the same time. Portable generators, which can be quite expensive, are purchased for these emergencies. Unlike major cities that have hospices in hospitals, most rural hospice's hands on care are primarily done in the home of the patient. Rural hospices payments are made on the same scale of hospices in metropolitan cities yet rural hospices face greater challenges. People born and raised in rural townships may not trust entering their loved ones in hospice as some compare them to nursing home care which can have a negative stigma; therefore it is very important for the hospice team to establish rapport as quickly as possible to assure the family that hospice is a safe and patient centered organization.

Chapter 5
Hospice in Hospitals

Some medical facilities have hospices within their walls or on their grounds. These hospices are necessary because some families do not have the assets and abilities to care for the dying patient. Though hospice is used by the young and old alike, many of the elderly are too frail and fragile to care for a dying member at home. Enrolling a family member in a hospital type hospice can take away some of the guilt and stress associated with care giving. Another reason for having viable hospital hospices is to assure the final needs of the dying are met as ethically and responsibly as when they were born.

Chapter 6
Respite Care

When caring for the dying person at home, caregivers are often neglecting their own health and welfare. It is a hospice requirement that a family member be present in the home to assist the person. Caring for the person day after day and watching the person suffer can be a devastating experience. For this reason, there is a respite care clause in the hospice contract when the person is dying at home. Respite allows a caregiver a much needed break from the daily routines of caring for the hospice patient. If the family asks for it and shows a need, the patient is transferred to a facility for up to 5 days allowing the family to get some rest and recuperation from the daily routines of care. After 5 days, the patient is transferred back to the home and hospice care is continued.

Chapter 7
Hospice Training

All team members undergo an extensive training program prior to being assigned to a hospice case. Volunteers must be at least 18 years of age and must show helpful and caring mental and physical aptitudes in order to be accepted for training. There is no specific gender requirement to serve although most of the volunteers are female. At least three out of ten volunteers drop out of training prior to completion because of the intense emotions associated with the training. The professional staff would rather see the volunteers drop out during the training phase rather than negatively affect the dying patient in real time. Hospice theories, lectures, dynamic one on one role plays, family counseling, videos and training film are all methods of conducting volunteer orientation and training. Listening skills are some of the most effective tools to use when working with dying patients. Listening is an art that many never learn. It requires actually hearing what the person is saying through words and body language and sometimes rephrasing those words. Patients relive their lives through the spoken word because their physical abilities decline as their bodies begin to shut down.

The hospice listener enhances the patient's entry into the shadow of death simply by being in their company. Reading books or newspapers to the dying soothes the patient in several ways. It reminds the patient that someone is in their presence. It also lets them feel that are still cared for. The dying patient can still hear and since they can hear, it is always advisable to not whisper or say anything harsh or negative around them. Hearing is usually the last sense to fade. (Callanan and Kelley, 36) One hospice volunteer remembered a patient asking if she wanted to go with her. The volunteer responded with, "I'll come later." These few words were helpful in allowing the patient to go on alone which she did peacefully. Solicitation of volunteers is done through newspaper and television advertising but most of the volunteer staff comes from former hospice patient families. Volunteers from these families are more attuned to the processes and spend more time as volunteers versus those who are just curious and think they want to serve. Facing death week after week is not something that all people readily adjust to. Those who do have the experience of working with people at the end of life provide one of the most rewarding services one human can offer another. That service is being there in body, mind and spirit. According to Miller, working with the dying helps one to see within themselves. (Miller and Cutshall, 2001)

Chapter 8
Hospice and Bereavement Therapy

Death does not end the relationship hospice has with the family because grieving is an individual process and takes time. Elisabeth Kubler-Ross in her book, <u>On Grief and Grieving,</u> (2005) reminds us that a grieving person goes through five stages of grief. These stages are denial, anger, bargaining, depression and acceptance. During the denial phase the survivor may think the death of the loved one is a dream and it really has not occurred. "There is a grace in denial" (Kubler-Ross, 10). When we receive news that is too painful to absorb, we use denial to protect ourselves. (Callanan and Kelley, 39) Family members have tendencies to say things around the patient to try to assure them that they are going to live. In reality, the family member is afraid to face the reality of death. The anger stage is expressed in several ways. Some survivors express anger that the person died without saying good bye. Anger may also be expressed at the dying or dead person because they did not care for themselves properly when they were living. There are instances where the survivor's anger stage is so intense that they refuse to attend the funeral of the deceased. During the bargaining

15

stage the survivor bargains with the Creator hoping that another chance will be given to the dying person and that their life will be spared. The survivor decides to attend church more often, pray a little more or treat others a little better. These changes in attitudes are seen as bargaining methods. When bargaining doesn't seem to work, the depression stage at some point in the survivor's life begins. During this stage it is very important that the survivor engages in a support system. This system may involve family members, the clergy or bereavement groups. If there are no clinically hindering processes going on with the survivor, acceptance of the death of the loved one finally takes place. Kubler-Ross indicates the grieving person does not have to go through these stages in any particular order. Hospice conducts bereavement sessions for family members at least once a month and more often if needed. Dying can be a consuming exercise for the patient and equally consuming for those caring for the patient. Oftentimes the health and welfare of caregivers are ignored during the course of caring for the dying. At the same time, stress and the normal pressures of life continue to increase. When the identified patient dies, the stress that's been building for months in the caregiver(s) escalates and has to be explored. The exploration of stress is a part of bereavement services provided by hospice. During the grieving period any bonds of affection to the deceased are gradually loosened. (Powell and Courtice, 212) It is during this loosening phase that the survivor requires the most assistance. This assistance often comes from friends, other relatives and the hospice bereavement team. If the reality of the loss is not accepted usually within a one to two year period, clinical and professional intervention may be necessary. There is no charge for the hospice bereavement groups and they are done as a community service. Although not intended to be, bereavement groups are seen as excellent avenues to use in recruiting volunteers.

Chapter 9
The Care Team

The hospice care team is typically made up of physicians, nurses, social workers, home health aides, ministers, nutritionists and volunteers. The most significant qualification for team members is to have and display a genuine care, concern and compassion for mankind. Each team member must understand that the dying person is still a person. There is a highly qualified licensed professional staff but most of the staff holds non- paying positions. Several of the volunteers come from backgrounds of having had a family member previously enrolled in a hospice program and see volunteering as a way to give back to the organization that which was given to their loved ones. Todd Michael in his book, The Evolution Angel, (Todd, 6) says, "Attending the death of another human being is awe inspiring and regarded as a sacred privilege of the highest order." A social worker's father died in his arms after suffering a heart attack. The death was sudden and unexpected. The reason the social worker gave for becoming a hospice volunteer was to hear how the dying communicated with their loved ones during their final days and hours before death. Though his father died in his arms, the father did not get a chance to say anything to his son before death appeared. Working with hospice became a catharsis for the social worker. A nurse volunteered because her mother was a former hospice patient and she was very pleased with the ways nursing and other staff treated her mother. She wanted to provide similar services to someone else. A fireman volunteered because his brother was in an auto accident and was cared for by a hospice team. He knew his brother did not suffer because of the care provided by the staff. He wanted to assist the hospice as a means of giving thanks for his brother's care. His volunteerism included setting up hospital beds for the patients and providing some transportation assistance as needed. Death is more of a surety than a good life although it is rarely discussed.

The introduction of hospice has helped society plan for death's arrival through advanced directives, living wills, and power of attorneys. These tools often assist the dying and the care givers to deal with the cumbersome nature of going into the unknown realm of life which is death.

Chapter 10
Family Interaction during the Transition

Family members enrolled in hospice past and present were interviewed in order to get some sense of their feelings and reactions to the death and dying of their relatives. (n=20) Families can be a cohesive group until a member becomes terminally ill. Regardless of the make up, educational or economic levels of this group, the thought of a member's death takes on a new set of attitudes and values. Members internalize the meaning of death and how it affects them personally. The birth order becomes more meaningful especially for the person who is next to the dying person either before they were born or after they were born. The question then becomes, "Am I next?" According to Powell and Courtice, "survivor guilt" is usually reserved for people who have outlived their peers or spouses. (Powell and Courtice, 214). Some families struggle with the health team when the physician announces that all means to heal the patient have been exhausted and hospice becomes an option for continuity of life care. Some families see the introduction of hospice as the sentence of death for their member. Financial questions concerning who is going to pay for the service come to the forefront. Questions about spirituality are raised and some even question the meaning of death. One of the greatest struggles families seem to experience is when a dying family member has HIV and AIDS. There are fewer visitors to the home when an AIDS patient is the identified dying member. There is a sense of shame expressed by the AIDS patient for having contracted the disease and bringing shame to the family. There is also a sense of anger expressed by some family members toward the dying AIDS patients for bringing shame to the family. Members who have had difficulty dealing with loss in the past tend to have greater difficulties working through current losses. Survivors of those dying with AIDS have few resources for mourning. (Worden, 141) The social worker plays a tremendous role in this area. He/she assists the family in working through past losses and they continue this care after the current loss. Some family members disagree with the type care the medical team provides the dying patient. There are those who want any and all medical and technical apparatus used to keep the patient alive as long as possible. Other family members who understand the expenses of care given to prolong the life of the patient disagree with those wanting life extended. Neither understands the pain and agony the dying patient experiences regardless of the medical treatment. Hospice workers are trained to assist the family in working out these differences. Hospice's interest lies in making the patient as pain free and dignified as possible during this final travel through the shadow of death. Because of the individualized care received by the hospice enrollee, there are some instances when a patient lives longer than the anticipated six month period. When this occurs, some hospices allow the patient to enter into palliative care. Others have the treating physician recertify the patient. When the patient begins again to show signs of physical and cognitive deterioration, they are re-enrolled in hospice. Interviews and surveys found families experiencing several different emotions when initial discussions were made concerning their family members entering a hospice care program. Entering hospice to some meant an order from the doctor that the patient was going to die soon. For this reason, many families fail to enter a patient into hospice until death is almost imminent. They don't realize that their family member could have lived a more peaceful and basically pain free end of life through hospice care. Death is something that individuals are reluctant to discuss openly. It's never an easy task even within the medical profession. Doctors are trained to heal but there is little training to deal with emotions associated with the loss of a patient. Physicians were sent a survey asking about their feelings on hospice. (n=10) The survey revealed that physicians don't do well when it comes to death and dying issues. They spend many years in medical school and are trained to care for patients and to affect a cure for their illnesses. David Keeler says medical professionals have been taught that death is the enemy. (Kessler, 10) Rarely is the physician taught to deal with the emotions of the dying patient. Dr. Daniel Tobin, in his book, "Peaceful Dying" says, "No where in my training was there formal instruction in caring for the dying." (Tobin, 6) Physicians struggle with their own immortality. The physician does not want to give up on the patient but realizes that some advanced stages of disease can not be cured. Psychologically, the physician is not giving up hope for the patient but after having treated the patient for a period of time and knowing there is no cure, he/she does not want to see their patient suffer with debilitating pain. He does want the patient to have comfort and a certain peace of mind. Once the patient is free of pain he/she can develop their own sense of hope. Whatever that sense of hope is for the patient, hospice is there for the rest of the patient's life to help them live out that hope.

Chapter 11
Traveling Through Hospice

David Kessler, in his book <u>The Needs of the Dying</u> says, "Death is a broad traveler in our society." (xvii) Death travels with us from the moment of birth and acts as a shadow until the last breath leaves the body. During the last six months of life of a terminally ill patient, the travel is made easier and more humanistic by enrolling the dying patient in a local and certified hospice organization.

After the treating physician has given a prognosis that curative medical treatment is no longer a viable option and death is likely to occur within six months a referral is made. With the patient and family's concurrence, the dying person may be enrolled in hospice. Enrolling does not negate his/her right to receive quality care from all providers. The patient does not give up any rights to refuse certain medications or certain forms of care. Every hospice care giver must respect the patient's rights to privacy whether in the home or in a hospital based hospice.

Chapter 12
Advanced Directives

Before and after a patient is enrolled in a hospice care program, it's important to complete advanced directives. If the family is not aware of the meanings and the reasons for advanced directives the social worker can assist in this process by acquiring the forms and assisting in the completion of the forms. Having (ADs) Advanced Directives completed and properly signed and DNR (Do Not Resuscitate) forms completed can assist the hospice team and the dying patient in many ways. If the DNR is not requested by the dying person when their cognitive abilities are intact, a family member may want the physician to try and resuscitate the patient. If the proper forms aren't signed family members may want life to be sustained as long as possible regardless of cost. Many families incur exorbitant medical costs long after their member has died because of failing to honor the dying person's wishes. Hospice is not there to treat the patient but to provide comfort and pain management support. A durable medical power of attorney signed by the dying person while their cognitive abilities are intact will allow someone who they have identified to legally make their wishes known when they are no longer able to communicate.

Chapter 13
Payment for Hospice Care

Hospice care is paid for by several sources. Most insurances cover hospice including Medicare and Medicaid. Donations are graciously accepted and are used to purchase durable medical equipment, medical supplies and transportation. Donations are also used to cover certain medications not directly related to the terminal illness and not covered by Medicare. Families of the deceased donate funds and equipment to hospices in memory of their loved ones. These donations are often lifeline additives for rural hospices. When the interdisciplinary care team has completed all assessments, intake forms, insurance forms and agreements, an empathetic holistic re-engagement with the patient's Source, his/her Divine, or his/her God begins. The hospice team facilitates and guides this engagement. During the reengagement with the Source, there are instances when the dying person appears to enter a new environment of happiness, Heaven or Nirvana. Kathleen Dowling Singh says, "Higher energies filter in." (Singh, 4) The patient shows a willingness to greet the hospice team members with a renewed sense of inner strength during the visits. The patient knows he/she is dying but with someone around them, they feel the visitor shares a piece of their heart. (Kubler-Ross, 167) The writer investigated the literature, conducted interviews and describes several of the visits with patients as hospice teams traveled with (cared for) the patients through the shadows of death. The names of the patients are disguised so that their earth identities remain sacred. The hospice team travels occurred with a variety of patients. (Appendix A)

Chapter 14
Dying and Communicating

Dying persons' requests are sometimes difficult to decipher. (Callanan and Kelley, 15)

The dying person has many signs of communicating with the survivors but the survivors often ignore these signs. Instances where the dying call out the name of someone who has already died is shrugged off as the patient's medications are causing them to hallucinate. When the dying person has that stare at one particular corner of the room and speaks to someone who is not seen by others, it is also attributed to the medications. In reality, the person is distancing him/herself from the outside environment and is entering the space of death or altered states of consciousness. The outer battle stills with the age of acceptance and with the sense of removal from the world in the person's psychological reality. (Singh, 197) Dying people often engage in early life memories and express these memories as if their psyche has traveled back in time. A ninety year old repeatedly called her mother's name and asked her to come and get her. She also spoke with people that were major figures in her early life. Singh says with the unleashing

of these past memories into consciousness, quite often we see ourselves with sometimes caustic clarity. (Singh, 200) Unfortunately,
some of these formerly repressed memories are negative in nature
and cause agitation in the dying patient. A seasoned hospice coun-
selor, minister or social worker can assist the family in dealing
with these memories, unleashing these memories helps the person
to relieve themselves of guilt.

Chapter 15
Challenges in Hospice Care

During hospice interventions, the team often encounters the unexpected. On one occasion the hospice nurse and social worker completely cleaned a patient's home after her death and prior to the arrival of the deceased siblings. When the patient became bedridden, she wanted the curtains to remain closed and the home dimly lit. She had small children but they were unable to clean the home as well as the mother during her healthier days. Hospice team members took turns doing housekeeping chores until the patient's death. When the family arrived for the funeral, they were pleased as to how well the sister had maintained her home. The extended family never knew that housekeeping was done by hospice. Team members never disclosed how the home had looked prior to their interventions. The thought of the possibilities of cleaning toilets, vacuuming, and other housekeeping duties is a reason some volunteers give for dropping out of hospice training. Hospice homemakers provide cleaning services in the patient's homes and run errands if a family member is not available. They are not in the home everyday but are there when the Hospice Registered Nurse deems their service appropriate. Volunteering is no place to bring or display middle class values. There is also no place for discrimination among the care provided any hospice patient. If any subtle discrimination based on race, sex, gender is noted during training sessions, the volunteer is not selected to serve. Volunteers are important members of the hospice team. They provide several of the services the dying person needs other than professional medical services. They may prepare food, wash clothing, read the Bible if the patient is religious oriented and has given permission to read. Religion is never introduced unless the patient or family member gives permission. There are patients who will ask the hospice team to pray for them. If this is done, the prayer should be referred to the Minister on the team. Praying for the recovery of the dying patient sends mixed signals and is inappropriate for the hospice team. Some forms of meditation may also assist the patient in diverting their concentration from pain to inner peace. Meditation helps the patient's mind to become still at the exclusion of all outside interferences. A person's culture, values, beliefs, and temperament will have an influence on which practice of prayer or meditation will be helpful. (Byock, 236)

Chapter 16
Pain and the Dying

When the patient is being treated by a physician, it is now a requirement to ask about the patient's pain levels. If there is no terminal illness or a progressive cancer; there is always the possibility of making the patient addictive to pain medications. When a person is dying, pain is never purely physical. (Byock, 214) The thoughts of loved ones being left behind and the thoughts of earthly chores left undone also inflict psychological pain in the dying. Doctors and the other hospice medical staff are tasked to do everything possible to relieve the patient's pain. In the dying patient, addiction is not a question to be explored. Pain relief is. Hospices have known families who show unreasonable concern about the dying family member becoming addicted to some of the powerful narcotic medications that terminal cancer can require. The concern should not be for the dying patient but for the survivors attending the patient. It is imperative that hospice along with some responsible family member control the pain medications from others.

Chapter 17
Holding On

Some dying patients want to hold on to life as long as they can. People who have been very active during their lives find it hard to become dependant on another person or agency. Hospice finds some of these patients to be passive resistant to their services.

Through time with these patients, the resistance is broken down. Through effective listening and communication by the staff, the dying person usually relinquishes his/her hold and accepts the services provided and accepts the fact that he is dying. After telling staff life stories and feeling assured they have been listened to, peace arrives. The dying person let go of that which was done in life and no longer has a need to be on top of the world. James E. Miller says, in One You Love is Dying, "this is their show, let them be the star." (6) There are some hospice patients who hold on to life because they have unfinished business to attend to. They may have bills that need to be paid and have not told the family about these bills. They may want to make amends with someone for having done something to that person in the past. They may not have seen a child or some of their children in many years and wait for those members to come to their bedsides for their last chats. It is during this holding on that the hospice team work closely with the family and prompts them to spend time with the dying member either in a group or alone. There are some dying patients who make confessions to the family before death. These are called "death bed confessions." Some of these confessions leave the survivors with psychic pain long after their family member has passed on. A family member of one family had been adopted and was never told this by the mother. He always assumed that he was just the only child of his mother and father. His mother confessed to him that he had been adopted. This death bed confession left the son bewildered and he entered therapy after the death of the mother. His need for therapy stemmed from his attachment to a parent. Catherine Sanders in her book, <u>Surviving Grief</u>, says, "Attachment becomes a fundamental form of completeness." (27) After being told that he was adopted by the dying mother his world became insecure. Without the knowledge that the son was adopted, hospice had no way of preparing him for this traumatic revelation. The attachment he had with his mother will again invoke any separation anxiety he may have experienced as a child. Babies attach to their mothers first and cry out in grief when separated from her. (Moody and Arcangel, 11)

Chapter 18
The End of the Journey

A mother goes through nine months of pregnancy and at the end of those nine months gives birth to a new baby. The baby enters this world in a helpless state after having come from another world. In that other world, the baby was protected, fed and cared for by some unseen Creator. After entering this world the baby is fed by a human, cuddled, touched and cared for so as not to become a marasmus baby. When he excretes, his/her diapers are changed and the infant enters a state of warmth and love. This physical touching while young translates to psychological touch as the child grows older. As a person enters the dying stages of life, he/she prepares to reenter that inner world from which he/she previously came from. During some hospice visits the dying person is seen lying in a fetal position. The dying entering an infant like state may become incontinent of urine and feces just the way he/she was as a baby. Just as the baby cried when the diaper was changed, the dying person often cries when the diaper is changed because he/she feels his dignity has been taken away. The hospice staff reminds the dying person that changing the diaper is a part of the care. Byock, in his book, "Dying Well" reminded a patient that an infant isn't undignified needing to be changed, and neither was he. (95)

Hospice for the patient, the family and the care team proves to be an enriching experience as each travels through the shadow of death using mind, body and spirit. No one ever travels alone because the journey begins at the moment of birth and everyone takes this journey. Some travel short distances as childhood illnesses take children through the shadow of death early on in life. Some travel and meet death through tragedies and families suffer because of the tragedies. There are those fortunate beings whose Creator gave them the chance to allow their families to make preparations for death. These are the ones who accepted entry into a hospice. In hospice the Creator makes the patient's pain less piercing by allowing the mind, body and spirit to work conjointly. This God allows a human being to share the heart of another and not get tired or seek rewards. This Creator allows a nurse to listen to the pace of the last heart beats of another. This is the God who created hospice, a team of caregivers who listens, who touch, who laugh, who cry, who travels with the patients and allows the dying to journey through the shadow of death and achieve holistic peace.

Chapter 19
When Death Occurs

When death occurs in a hospital setting the attending physician usually pronounces the death of the patient. When the patient is enrolled in hospice at home, there are specific guidelines that must be agreed upon prior to the family member's enrollment. There are members who want to contact emergency services when a change in the person's condition is noted and not understood. Families are briefed that if they feel that imminent death is occurring or they feel the person has died, they are instructed not to call 911 but to notify the hospice staff. Eva Shaw in her book, <u>What to Do When a Loved One Dies,</u> quotes Dr. Fred Jordan who says, "Most people are pronounced dead when heart and lung functions cease. Brain death requires documentation by special equipment generally only available in a hospital setting." (6) The hospice staff will contact the physician who will pronounce the time of the patient's death. The staff will contact the funeral home that the family identifies as the one the deceased member is to be transferred to.

When the person dies it becomes a very emotional and sometimes difficult time for the family. Decisions have to be made about funeral arrangements, care of the deceased assets and belongings. The hospice social worker is available to assist the survivors work through these processes.

The research showed how hospice services in the home gave a holistic meaning to death and dying by monitoring the body, mind and spirit of the dying person in a home environment in contrast to dying in a sterile hospital setting. Compassionate care exists around the clock in the patient's home when hospice is involved. Hospice and all the care and services provided psychically takes the family structure back in time when family members died at home and the casket remained in the home until the funeral.

Hospitals are oftentimes used to sustain a person's life and can become a testament to the power of the shadow world. (Kaufman, 296) Hospice care done in the patient's home uses the holistic approach and travels with the patient through this shadow of death. Hospice in the dying patient's home was also found to be the best holistic approach for the individual to peacefully reenter into the world from whence he/she came. The spirit world.

Works Cited

Buchwald, Art. <u>Too Soon to Say Goodbye</u>. New York: Random House, 2006.

Byock, Ira. <u>Dying Well</u>. New York: The Berkley Publishing Group, 1997.

Callanan, Maggie and Kelley, Patricia. <u>Final Gifts</u>. New York: Bantam, 1992

Kaufman, Sharon R. <u>And a Time to Die</u>. New York: Simon & Shuster, 2005.

Keesler, David. <u>The Needs of the Dying</u>. New York: Harper, 2007.

Michael, Todd. <u>The Evolution Angel</u>. New York: The Penguin Group, 2008.

Miller, James E. <u>How Can I Help?</u> Indiana: Willowgreen, 2000.

---, ed. <u>One You Love Is Dying</u>. Indiana: Willowgreen, 1997.

Moody, Raymond Jr. and Dianne Archangel. <u>Life After Loss</u>. New York: HarperCollins, 2001.

Powell, Leslie S. and Courtice, Katie. <u>Alzheimer's Disease, A Guide for Families</u>. Massachusetts: Addison-Wesley, 1983.

Salzberg, Sharon. <u>The Kindness Handbook</u>. Colorado: Sound-strue, 2008.

Sanders, Catherine M. <u>Surviving Grief</u>. New York: Wiley &
Sons, 1992.

Shaw, Eva. <u>What To Do When A Loved One Dies</u>. California:
Dickens Press, 1994.

Singh, Kathleen D. <u>The Grace in Dying</u>. New York: Harper-
Collins, 2000.

Tobin, Daniel R. <u>Peaceful Dying</u>. Massachusetts: Persus, 1999.

Worden, J. William. <u>Grief Counseling and Grief Therapy 3rd
edition</u>. New York:

Springer, 2002.

Appendix A

The Minister

Ms. Banes was a young recently ordained minister. She was a college graduate, a musician, and the love of her mother and father. She was one of four children but the only minister in the family. During her days with hospice, she taught Biblical passages and even gave verbal tests on follow-up visits. Although the visits were always warm, there were days when team members felt as if they were back in school during the patient's Biblical tests. There were days when she struggled with pain but still managed to read passages from the Bible. When she became weak to the point of being unable to read, she pointed to the Bible during the visits and the team took turns reading and discussing passages and meanings of the verses. The team's readings diverted the thoughts of her pain as there were hardly any grimacing signs displayed by her during the process. Upon her death, her mother and father donated furniture to the Hospice organization on behalf of their daughter. The only stipulation was that a Bible be placed on the conference table for others to learn that hospice is a God caring organization.

The Angel Child

Little Baby Maggie was a four year old with a rare disease that restricted the control of her muscular movements, her speech, and eye movements. She was physically transferred from her mother's lap to the bed and was assisted in all her activities of daily living. When first introduced to the little Angel, she responded with the most beautiful smile that any compassionate teary eyed practitioner could see. When any team member talked with her, those bright eyes moved horizontally in rapid succession. Although she did not speak verbally, her mother taught her to communicate with friends and neighbors by blowing kisses. This she performed eagerly until the progression of the disease took its toll. When this occurred, she could no longer raise her little arms. The disease would not allow for any weight gain and though she was four years old, she weighed less than 50 pounds. Her fragile little body never dampened her delight to see a hospice team member. Hospice was fortunate enough to be care givers for her during her last birthday.

The team gave a birthday party with cake and all the trimmings. During the travel with this precious child through the shadow, her facial expressions showed no fear. The outer glow of her persona reminded everyone that she was only on loan to the earth world and she knew where her spirit was headed. Volunteers swore that her brittle little collar bones resembled little wings. During the day of her funeral, there were overcast skies during the early morning hours and a threat of rain. When her miniature pretty pink casket was carried from the church to the grave site, the sun came out brightly and the clouds slowly disappeared. Later that day, heavy rains soaked the town. This confirmed the conviction that all had been in the presence of an Angel.

The soldier's wife

Ms. Jenkins lost her husband through death many years before she entered into hospice. Her children worked during the day and Hospice visits to her was like making new friends and having someone to talk to. Her travel through the shadow involved bringing out all the photo albums of her and the husband when they were younger. He had been in World War II and she was proud of him having served the country. During each visit, she presented a different piece of memorabilia and explained when and where it originated. She knew the times of the team's visits and waited patiently at the door. If during a visit someone arrived a bit late," she would say, "I was waiting on you." "I thought you weren't coming to see me today." The travels showed her life as a young lady, a wife, and a mother. Her original home and childhood was in a different country. She said they moved to the United States because of the increased opportunities afforded them. Her journey ended with her showing the flag presented at her husband's funeral many years earlier. After showing the last page of her photo album and the flag presented to her during the husband's funeral, she gradually became too weak to greet the care team at the door. Her family began medical leave from their job and assisted hospice in the final days. Her final act was to give the team a coin shown during the journey. To her the coin symbolized the beginning and the end of life as she had lived it which was expressed earlier on during hospice care.

Mr. Parker

Mr. Parker was a proud southerner who drank at least two colas each day. He also smoked cigars most of his adult life but quit after being diagnosed with lung cancer. He proudly talked about the old south and the many accomplishments of his life. He was a former member of the city council and former Mayor of the town. He looked forward to the visits and always offered a cola to the hospice team. There were times when no cola was wanted by a caregiver but it made him feel better to know that he was sharing one of his favorite pastimes with someone. To him, sharing a cola meant accepting his friendship. During this gentleman's travel through the shadow, he lost his physical mobility and was no longer able to venture outside the home. The hospice team took a video of the city and some of the places he previously traveled.

The video was brought back to the home and a video player was set up in his room. He expressed gratitude to the hospice team for being so sensitive to his needs. Each day until his death and through the use of the video, he mentally went out on the town, cola in hand, reliving the scenes of his life. He celebrated life through the end of his life and hospice played a role in the celebration.

Mrs. Hinson

Mrs. Hinson was a heavy smoker practically all her adult life. Her husband of over forty years indicated to the hospice team that she previously predicted one day her life would be shortened by some type lung disease because she smoked so many cigarettes. Ironically, she quit smoking the day of her lung cancer diagnosis but it was too late. Mrs. Hinson insisted that the hospice team member(s) attending her on any given day stay for lunch or dinner. Knowing this, the member scheduled to see her was expected to carry an appetite along with their caring attitudes. Mrs. Hinson started a no smoking campaign during her illness and was so successful in her efforts that the two hospice staff that were smokers quit and started their own no-smoking campaigns. Her travels through the shadow were heroic for she extended the lives of so many others through her "quit smoking" lectures.

Mr. Clifton

Mr. Clifton lived in the rural in a wooden house that needed several repairs. He admitted he could not afford the repairs because of the medical bills associated with his care. It was a hospice requirement to have a phone for contacts but this he could not afford. A phone was installed by the hospice organization and some minor repairs were made to the home by volunteers. Though the gentleman was on his final journey, he made feeble attempts to assist in the home's repairs but the team insisted that he take it easy and get much needed rest. Though he lived a simple life, he treasured a rose garden in the yard and indicated the rose garden was started years ago as a memorial to his deceased wife. He said the rose garden always reminded him of how he could make something pretty out of a sticky situation. His final request was to have a bouquet of the roses placed on his grave after his death. After hearing his final request, the hospice team began to nurture his rose garden right along with his care. During each visit, the garden was watered and weeded by a team member and the roses grew even more beautifully. Upon his death, full bouquets of the roses were placed on his casket.

Mr. Stanley

Mr. Stanley was a minister and outstanding member of the church community. He was an inspiration to the community in which he lived and was very instrumental in steering the kids away from drugs. A stroke brought him down from the pulpit of the church but this did not dampen his spirits from keeping the kids off drugs. When he enrolled in hospice, a nurse assigned to his care discovered that he was the mentor who influenced her to stay in school. She gave an account of having grown up in a drug infested area of town but was made to attend church by her parents. A sermon by this minister had stuck with her for years. He often preached you can get yourself out of the pits of hell if you let God lead you. This was part of her inspiration in becoming a nurse and moving away from her childhood environment. Now was her opportunity to pay him back by traveling with him through the shadow. During her visits, she constantly reminded him of the influence he had on her life. Oh what joy he showed each time she came to visit. The nurse was with him as he took his final breath. She indicated his circle will now be unbroken for his spirit will live within her.

Ms. Jackson

In another instance the mother, Ms. Jackson was the hospice patient. She had five adult children and each lived in different states. The oldest sibling had not spoken to the youngest brother in over 20 years because of his chronic drug abuse. It was clearly evident to the social worker that much bitterness existed among all the siblings. Since they lived in different states, they rarely visited the mother within the same time frames. The dying mother pleaded with the children to try and get along with each other. The Social Worker conducted several group sessions which ended with the older sibling and the younger brother finally hugging and promising their mother that things would get better. With that promise, the shadow disappeared and the mother experienced a long sought after peace. When a hospice patient holds on after all physical symptoms of life seem to fade away, there is usually some unfinished earthly or psychosocial business the patient is dealing with. The hospice team counsels family members about the possibility of this unfinished business and request that they make individual visits with the dying member. In most instances after these individual visits are made, the patient will let go and travel peacefully into the shadow. On this occasion, the visits by the children and their evidence of making amends were enough to satisfy their mother. These acts were acts of sympathetic Joy. (Salzberg, 30). Shortly after she saw that the children were going to be alright, she died.

Mr. Donald

One very difficult intervention occurred when a young married male patient with three children insisted his wife promise not to marry again after his death. The wife was willing to make this vow for the husband to die in peace but felt the husband's siblings prompted him to make this request. Her children, who were more progressive thinkers than their aunts and uncles, cautioned the mother about making this commitment. The patient's siblings also made subtle suggestions for the wife to make this commitment.

This created friction among the family clan which prompted several sidebar discussions. There were many social worker and chaplain counseling sessions with this family. The numerous interventions were meant to prolong the agony of making a decision by the wife. Although hospice services were done primarily in the home, the patient had a medical crisis and all the siblings insisted he be taken to the hospital even if it required leaving Hospice care. The patient died on the way to the hospital. The promise not to remarry was never made or the promise was broken. His wife remarried after three years had past.

Ms. Harvey

Ms. Harvey worked in real estate and met a social worker during his transfer to the small community. The worker rented a house through the agency and prepaid two month's rent prior to his arrival. Ms. Harvey welcomed the new comer and thought he should be refunded one month's rent because he arrived before the first month's rent was due. She contacted the head of the agency who disagreed with the refund. Ms. Harvey apologized and told the social worker she thought this was unfair. She hoped that this act would not taint the worker's image of the community. The social worker was one of the key players in starting a hospice in the small town. After hospice got started and ten years later, Ms. Harvey was stricken with a terminal illness and was enrolled in hospice. The social worker who she met ten years earlier, who she thought had been treated unfairly, became one of her hospice care givers. She felt at ease during her care and remembered the day of his arrival. The worker visited at least once a week and read to her when she no longer was able to read. She was very fond of the Bible and her faith was strong. The irony of her story was that she was the first to greet the social worker upon his arrival in the town and he was the last person to say goodbye to her before her travel ended.

Me Ma

Me Ma was a sweet lady of 90 years who had raised eight children. All were alive except her oldest son who had passed away seven years earlier. This son had taken the place of his father whose death occurred twenty years earlier. He took his mother fishing and became the maintenance man for her home because she lived alone. After the son's unexpected death, Me Ma's health began to gradually decline. Her granddaughter had a 3 year old son who had never seen his great grandmother (Me Ma) until he and his mother moved from California to Me Ma's home town. The little boy immediately showed a special interest in his great grandmother. He went to her each time he was in her presence without being prompted. He talked with her and gave big smiles and hugs. He often conducted conversations with her that seemed somewhat gibberish to other listeners but the hospice team sensed that Me Ma understood. The family thought the child's behavior was loving but odd. They began to say the 3 year old was a reincarnated soul. They thought he could possibly be the reincarnated soul of his great grandfather, Me Ma's husband. When Me Ma became bed ridden the little boy stayed by her bedside as much as possible. When his cousins came over to play, he refused and stayed at the bedside of his Me Ma. The hospice team and the family praised the little boy for he brought a smile to Me Ma's face when no one else could. When Me Ma passed away, the little boy was there and went to the bed to hold her hand one last time. He was taken aside and told that Me Ma would not be with him anymore because God needed her and she was gone to Heaven. The child asked about Heaven and was told stories of where it was located and how one gets to go there. The child may not understand all the adults are going through but even a limited understanding is important. (Kubler-Ross, 160).

Ms. Joseph

Ms. Joseph was a high school teacher and a highly respected member of the community. She and her husband lived alone and both had looked forward to retiring in a few years but cancer forced an early retirement on her. She enrolled in hospice and received care in the home. During her teaching years, she carried a seemingly happy demeanor. She was a somewhat robust lady with a few friends. Cancer reduced her body to a very small frame. It was difficult for her to show pictures of herself as she looked in the classroom a few months earlier compared to the size of her present physical state. She spoke of the different kids in her classes and made mention of those who had become highly successful in their own right. Sadness on her face seemed more intense when she discussed the infrequent visits of close friends during the final weeks of life. Some of her friends called and promised to visit but rarely kept their promise. Daniel R. Tobin, M.D. indicates family and friends who love you can be comforting to the dying person. (Tobin, 52). Some people want to remember the dying person in the physical form as they were in their normal life. Hospice became a sounding board for this teacher because the thoughts of dying alone depressed her. She became very angry and displayed this by showing hostility towards some of the team members. Art Buchwald says, "The worst thing about depression is the anger that goes with it." (Buchwald, 38). Social Workers and ministers play valuable roles when signs of depression appear in the patients. They are trained to assess and assist the patient in working through the anger. This patient did not have time to work through all the anger within her. Though hospice workers were with her through the journey, peace for her did not come easily.

Mr. Jeffrey

The final journey was with Mr. Jeffrey, the comedian. For years he was a comedian on a Saturday morning children's television show and he loved entertaining. When he was diagnosed with cancer, he went through radiation treatment, chemotherapy and clinical trials but none of these dampened his comedy or his spirits. He carried a one man comedy show to each place where he received treatment and it was especially welcomed on the cancer wards. Some of his favorite jokes were about the bald head that the chemo therapy left him with. The team never met a patient with such external joy and he spread this joy to every person he met. His final stage play was with the hospice team. If impending death made him sad, he covered it easily with his comedy at first. He entertained the hospice team with different tales of humor with each visit. Caring for him was payment for the free concerts he gave at his home. He could rattle off lines of some of the more famous comedians and never repeat a single joke. Finally, his curtain calls began to come fewer and fewer and he became a bed ridden patient. When his breathing became more difficult, his comedy and laughter turned to tears. As his days grew shorter, each hospice visit saw more and more tears from his eyes. One day a team member told one of his jokes; he stopped crying, smiled, took one last breath and exited this life.

Appendix B

Please circle your responses after each question. Responses are for statistical purposes and results will be used as part of a Doctoral Dissertation. Please do not sign the form or indicate your name. Your assistance is appreciated.

Family survey

1. Please choose one of the following to indicate the reason you enrolled your family member in Hospice;
   ( ) I heard the services were free.
   ( ) I have hospice on my insurance.
   ( ) I had a relative enrolled in Hospice in the past.

2. What do you expect the hospice team to provide your family member?
   ( ) quality care
   ( ) pain medication
   ( ) housekeeping
   ( ) companionship

3. If you were diagnosed with a terminal illness with a death expectancy of six months or less, where would you prefer to die?
   ( ) nursing home
   ( ) hospital
   ( ) home with family

4. Should spirituality be a part of hospice care?
   ( ) yes
   ( ) no
   ( ) I don't care to respond to this.

5. Would you be willing to volunteer any of your time to hospice?
   ( ) yes
   ( ) no
   ( ) maybe

Thank you for your responses

Please circle your responses after each question. Responses are for statistical purposes and results will be used as part of a Doctoral Dissertation. Please do not sign the form or indicate your name. Your assistance is appreciated. Thank you.

Physician/Nurse Survey

1. As a Provider, what are your feelings when you've done all you can for your patient and realize nothing more can be done to help the patient survive?
   (a) Sadness
   (b) Joy
   (c) a sense of loss as a Provider
   (d) a sense of relief that my patient won't have to suffer any longer.
   (e) I'm ambivalent.

2. Do you believe that death is the final form of a person's life?
   (a) Yes
   (b) No
   (c) I don't care to respond to this question.

3. If you had the chance to provide at least one hour a week of unpaid care to a hospice patient, would you agree to do so?
   (a) Yes
   (b) No
   (c) I don't have time.
   (d) I don't care to respond to this question.

4. If you were a patient with a terminal illness and a short life expectancy, where would you prefer to die?
   (a) Hospital
   (b) nursing home
   (c) in my own home
   (d) in the home of a relative or friend.

5. In my practice, a family should be told that the patient is dying by;
   (a) The physician
   (b) the nurse
   (c) the minister
   (d) the social worker
   (e) should not be told.

6. Do you believe the family should be provided counseling by the hospice staff after the family member's death?
   (a) Yes
   (b) No
   (c) this should be the family's decision.

7. Should every hospital have a hospice staff?
   (a) Yes
   (b) No
   (c) It depends on the hospital's budget.

8. Were you provided training on hospice care in medical school or nursing school?
   (a) Yes
   (b) No
   (c) very little.

Volunteer questionnaire
1. Have you had any experience working with dying patients?
   (yes)
   (no)

2. Please indicate one of these as your highest reason for volunteering.
   (a) I want to learn about death and dying.
   (b) (b) I had a family in hospice.
   (c) (c) I'm doing a study on death and dying.

3. Have you ever witnessed a person dying of cancer?
   (a) Yes
   (b) no

4. Have you ever attended to a person dying of cancer?
   (a) yes
   (b) no

5. Would you be able to work with and visit an AIDS patient?
   (a) yes
   (b) no

6. Would you be willing and able to travel through rural areas?
   (a) Yes
   (b) no
   (c) I'm not sure.

Thank you for your responses.